HOW TO GET INTO KETOSIS IN 24 HOURS

10 STEPS TO SAFETY

Jennifer J Collins

*I want to dedicate this book to all those who have supported us
during all this year, especially to my dear and beloved family.*

*Dedicate it to all my friend and to all of you who acquired this
book,*

*I hope that all the information in this work will be of great help
to all of you, that all your goals and objectives will be achieved and
that you will look better every day, with the quality of life that you
deserve.*

*Do not forget that you are a unique person and do not care what
people tell you,
you have a lot of courage.*

INTRODUCCIÓN

It can usually take your body 2-7 days to go into ketosis depending on your body type, your level of physical activity, and what you eat. You can wait the 7 days or you can follow these 10 steps to get into ketosis as quickly as possible.

Also, if you accidentally break the Keto diet this iBook will help you get into ketosis quickly.

I want to be the person who helps you feel good about yourself the most, I was in your shoes and I understand that perfectly, one day you will help me to improve my health and be spectacular.

I want you to experience this pleasant feeling of feeling better about yourself in all aspects. Also, if you accidentally break the Keto diet this iBook will help you get into ketosis quickly.

GRATTITUDE

◆ ◆ ◆

Of all the recipes for achieving abundance and prosperity in our lives, the best we can practice is gratitude.

Because feeling a sincere gratitude for what you have automatically and if effort, rather be to your life,

That's why it's so important for you to start now to value and recognize all the blessings you've already received.

Even if you cannot see it physically yet, that is why I am going to express here my gratitude that I have long expressed every morning when I got up and that has allowed me to be more grateful and to stay in the frequency of daily abundance and prosperity.

Being grateful brings me benefit when I close my eyes and expressed with sincerity, really feeling the gratitude in your heart.

Knowing that the creator God of the universe is conspiring to give you what you desire.

Dear God thank you for this day, I thank you for allowing me to experience this magical moment in my life.

Thank you for my family for my friends and my loved ones. Thank you for my health and well-being. For all the functions of my body that are performed to perfection.

Thank you for my house and everything in it. Thank you for all my possessions and for my home aspect of my life.

Thanks,

Because I appreciate all that I am today. For the morning sun, for the birds singing and the flowers in the morning.

Thank you for all the beauty that surrounds me at this time. Thank you for the prosperity I receive and will receive multiplied.

Thanks for every smile I will see and receive today. For all the blessings I will enjoy today.

For the opportunities that are unfolding before me. I choose to radiate gratitude to everyone and do everything I contacted today.

My heart is filled with recognition and thanksgiving for all you have given me and for the opportunity to help many people achieve happiness and feel better every day.

My God, thank you for opening my heart. Thank you for the wonderful gift again.

My God, thank you for the wonderful gift of my life.

Jennifer J Collins

WHAT IS INTERMITTENT FASTING?

Why does it help you lose weight?

How about the idea of fasting without putting too much effort into it? Everything you need to know about intermittent fasting.

Intermitten t Fasting, or IFA, is the most popular weight loss program today, and many celebrities, such as Hugh Jackman, Chris Hemsworth, and even Benedict Cumberbatch, have jumped on the Intermittent Fasting bandwagon.
And Bing's doctor in Raw, a primary care physician, said he lost 100 pounds (ca. 45 kg) in just 18 months thanks to Intermittent Fasting.

Before he tried the technique he weighed 300 pounds (0.14 t), so it seems that intermittent fasting is a real miracle.

What is the secret behind it that makes it so effective? Let's unravel the truth of this weight loss madness with a question that lingers in our minds.

Is it possible that the human body can endure long hours without food daily? Let's investigate a little first who created intermittent fasting.

In general, it is an ancient practice but it has nothing to do with your dream of achieving a perfect body to go to the beach in fact, humans have done things like that all their lives.

Important Greek personalities such as Pythagoras, Socrates and Plato helped to purify their spirit and mind.

Some major religions practice fasting to strengthen their faith. Mahatma Gandhi, fasting 17 times during his campaigns for India's independence, not only lost a few pounds but also overthrew the British government.

But when fasting gained recognition as a means of losing weight was popularized by the American writer Upton Sinclair, in the 20th century he practiced juice cleanliness and fasting simultaneously.

In August 2012 fasting gained recognition from the health and fitness community thanks to the influence of doctor and journalist Michael Moss Lee, he published a book on the subject in January 2013 entitled the fasting diet.

Before we continue we need to clear up misconceptions about this technique.

Firstly, intermittent fasting is often considered to be a type of diet, with intermittent fasting you do not control what you eat but take care when you do.

It is not a diet plan but a feeding pattern, we will explain this later in detail, for now, let's move on to the next myth of intermittent fasting.

The second misconception about this practice is that you must starve yourself, if we look in the dictionary for the meaning of hungry we'll read; "Intense and prolonged food shortage" on the other hand fasting means; "Total or partial deprivation of food for a while"

With him there you still have to eat and drink but it must be in a limited time.

That's why intermittent fasting is also considered a restricted feeding.

In time the third and final mistake that prevents health enthusiasts from trying this controversial weight loss program is the safety and well-being problems associated with intermittent fasting.
Let's get to the bottom of this by discussing how this technique works.

We mentioned earlier that intermittent fasting is a pattern of eating with fasting your entire day or week divided into two parts.

The feeding period and the fasting period, during the feeding period you can eat a regular meal, so if you don't need to starve.

During the fasting period you are not allowed to eat any food. No! Not a single bite can touch your lips.

But there is an exception to this rule during the fasting period you can drink but only water, tea or coffee without sugar or cream, please.
In some cases you can eat hundreds of calories or a combo of fruits and vegetables while you are in fasting mode.

How can you divide your day or week into a meal period and a fasting period?

Can it be 2 hours of fasting and 22 hours of eating? It doesn't work like that, that's not an intermittent fast. That's compulsive eating.

The eating patterns you can follow are the 16-8 pattern, also known as "leangains" which was invented by fitness expert Martin Beckham "leangains" is an ideal fasting schedule for beginners, no kidding.

This method involves fasting for 14-16 hours per day, the remaining 6-8 hours are for the feeding period. The 5:2 pattern "the fasting diet" method created by British physician and journalist Michael Mosley if the same subject who revived the popularity of intermittent fasting.

This is lighter than the "leangains" protocol because you can eat 500 to 600 calories or high-calorie foods during the 2 days of fasting. And then you can eat naturally for 5 days. "Eat Stop

Eat was created by fitness expert Brad Bailey with this intermittent fasting eating pattern, you have to fast for 24 hours.

Once or twice a week for example you can start your fast on Monday at 12 pm and it will end on Tuesday the next day at 12 pm.

Alternating day fasting as the name suggests is when you fast every day and a half is a fasting period in a fasting period you can eat 500 to 600 calories or nothing at all.

The Warrior Diet It was popularized by fitness expert Ori Hofmekler this method requires fasting all day.

You can still eat small portions of fruits and vegetables. The feeding period is from 6 pm to 10 pm and you can eat a large meal.

The main concern about intermittent fasting is the large amount of time required for the fasting period. We are scheduled to eat breakfast, lunch, dinner, and a couple of snacks throughout the day.

How would your body feel if you skipped any of these meals? You may experience hunger, weakness, dizziness, or vomiting. You may also have sudden mood swings.
 How to go from frustration to irritation are normal bodily reactions during the first few weeks or months of fasting.

That's because the body is still adjusting to the new regimen. What can fasting really accomplish? Over time your body will eventually overcome the side effects, under normal circumstances your body gets energy from the food you eat. This is stored in your liver and muscles.

What about when you are fasting? Your body gets fuel from its last reserve.

The stored fats are burned to become energy the longer you fast, the more fat will be burned in the process.

What are the other health benefits of this technique besides helping your body get rid of unwanted pounds?

Good,
 > Can prevent type 2 diabetes
> Promote insulin resistance
> Good for the heart, may prevent cancer
> Improves brain function
> It promotes longevity and simplifies your lifestyle.

Because you don't have to plan to cook or pack 3-6 meals a day you can save money and time when shopping and preparing food. Hey! That means fewer dishes to wash up too.

Although intermittent fasting looks promising, this weight loss solution is not for everyone. If you really want to try the technique, we suggest that you consult your doctor first.
 Especially in these cases; Diabetes low blood pressure Pregnancy or attempted pregnancy History of eating disorders.

In addition, children and adolescents are advised not to try fasting, because at this stage of their development they need more energy than adults. You must also remember that you cannot lose weight through intermittent fasting alone.

Because you are always fasting, your body needs adequate nutrition from healthy foods such as dairy, lean protein, nuts and seeds, vegetables, whole grains, and whole and unprocessed foods.

It's also safe to exercise while fasting, but we recommend exercising after your body has adjusted and you don't have any side effects such as hunger or weakness. It's hard to lose weight no matter what weight loss program you choose - sacrifices have to be made.

Saying goodbye to your favorite fatty foods or not eating at all once in a while. Keep in mind that you should check with your doctor before starting any activity - intermittent fasting may work for others but may not be right for you. It's not because you can't keep away from that bag and you're either not self-controlled enough.

It may have something to do with your body's constitution - don't despair - there are other weight loss programs besides intermittent fasting that you can mix and match like the Keto diet.

THE INTERMITTENT FASTING

◆ ◆ ◆

We love intermittent fasting here I will show you 10 mistakes that people often make and that you should know.

The intermittent fasting for an easy way together with the Keto diet to lose weight without difficulties, but there are several mistakes you can make when doing the intermittent fasting.

"Intermittent fasting consists of establishing more specific time intervals for meals and between 12 and 16 hours of fasting per day", intermittent or sporadic fasting are more common daily (at least 12 hours of fasting, the best known pattern being "16/8"), there are others, such as weekly (usually one or two days a week of fasting, followed or not). Within this second option, the most popular is the so-called "5:2 diet", which advocates eating normally five days a week and a severe reduction in intake (over 75%) the next two. Fasting on a monthly basis (fasting a couple of days in a row each month) is practiced to a lesser extent.

KETOGENIC DIET

◆ ◆ ◆

It's very fashionable these days if you've heard of the ketogenic diet or "Keto", as it's known in English. It's become very popular over the last few years.

There are more and more publications about it, and the interest on the internet is very high.   But what exactly is the ketogenic diet?

What does ketogenic mean, to begin with? And how is it done? In this course you will learn everything you need to know about it.

First, let's get something straight. What does the word "ketogenic" mean?

Basically, it has to do with the fact that the body can function on two types of fuels.

One is the sugar in the carbohydrates in the food we eat, which is the main fuel used by most people today.

For example, when you eat bread, pasta, rice, potatoes, etc. The other fuel is fat. The ketogenic diet is a very low carbohydrate diet.

So low in carbohydrates, the body has to switch to using fat as the main fuel.

For example, fat from natural foods such as eggs, meat, avocados, butter, olive oil, nuts, etc.

Even the brain can get energy from fats. When the body runs out of sugar, the liver converts the fat into energy molecules called ketones, which provide the brain with energy.

And the diet that allows this is called ketogenic, since it produces ketones.

This is where the name of this type of diet comes from. Obtaining energy mainly from fat, a state known as "ketosis", has many benefits.

For example, it turns you into a fat-burning machine. In this state you lose weight without going hungry because you burn fat all the time, even when you sleep. And because it gives you enormous amounts of energy.

As to why the ketogenic diet has become super popular in recent years: It's really nothing new.

Its foundations have been built up over a long period of time. It's a strict low ketogenic, gluten-free diet, and it's similar to the Paleolithic diet.

It also looks a lot like the old, well-known Atkins diet. The basic idea is basic, and is that it is based on natural foods, simply avoid foods; such as sugar, fast and processed foods, bread, pasta, rice, etc.

Instead, you eat meat, fish, eggs, vegetables and natural fats, such as butter.

What's different about the ketogenic diet? That it is an ultra-improved low ketogenic diet, from which you can be sure you will get maximum benefits.

We'll get to the details later.

But, as I was saying, the ketogenic diet is an ultra-improved version of an old idea.

Similar diets have been tried for decades, even centuries. These similar diets are becoming increasingly well known because they work.

This might have an evolutionary explanation, since our ancestors didn't eat refined foods, or sugar the way we do today; so our bodies may not be adapted to those foods. Modern science shows that it works.
  On a ketogenic diet, most people can lose excess weight without going hungry, and multiple health problems, such as insulin resistance, diabetes, or obesity, among others, tend to improve.

Most importantly, the ketogenic diet is not just used as a temporary solution.

Many people enjoy it as a lasting lifestyle.

Not just for weight loss, but for long-term health and well-being and for staying in shape all year round.

Many people feel energetic, full of energy and lucidity, and have stable blood sugar levels.

Hunger disappears, cravings for sweet foods are reduced, so there's no need to be eating frequently anymore.

Time is saved by being satisfied with fewer meals per day. You eat delicious food every time you are hungry, and you don't even have to count calories.

Most people feel so full on the ketogenic diet that they can eat every time they are hungry, and still eat less and reduce excess weight.

1 STEP

EAT LESS THAN 20 GRAMS OF CARBOHYDRATES A DAY.

◆ ◆ ◆

To get into ketosis quickly, you need to dramatically reduce the way and the amount you eat carbohydrates.

Check your intake to 50 grams per day if you want to go into ketosis faster reduce your carbohydrate intake below 50 grams per day.

That can be very difficult if it's your first time on the ketogenic diet and if you were eating a lot of high-sugar carbohydrates.

This is why it is not advisable to eliminate them completely from one moment to the next but to gradually reduce their consumption.

If you are considering starting the ketogenic diet, the least you can do is change your carbohydrate intake by eating less and less and changing the form.

Most people believe that eating carbohydrates is only possible through pasta, rice and grains.

But not many vegetables and fruits are basically carbohydrates - fruits like oranges and vegetables like sweet potatoes are high in carbohydrates and you don't gain anything by substituting one serving of rice for another from Dad because they are the same in terms of their macronutrient content.

The carbohydrates you should start eating are green leafy vegetables like broccoli, cabbage, cauliflower, lettuce and spinach.

These foods, besides being healthier, contain fewer carbohydrates, which allow your body to release the excess glucose that carbohydrates provide and prepare it for ketosis.

Once you have managed to reduce your carbohydrate intake you are ready to enter the ketogenic diet.

To achieve ketosis quickly try to limit your carbohydrate intake to less than 20 grams per day and increase your good fats to a large extent.

Similarly, protein should be reduced by 25% this is calculated based on your weight of 0.8 and one gram of protein per kilogram of body weight.

By reducing your carbohydrates extremely and moderating the protein while increasing the consumption of fat your body will be ready to start ketosis.

2 STEP

DO A FATTY FAST OR A COMBINED FAST WITH INTERMITTENT FASTING

◆ ◆ ◆

Intermittent fasting is a perfect way to support and accelerate your ketosis process once you start the ketogenic diet. Keep fasting from the last meal of the previous day and open your 8-hour feeding window past noon.

In this way you will be forcing your body to take all the energy from the glucose you consumed the day before by consuming it more quickly.

So, when you break the fast and your body will have no choice but to lead to the process of ketosis, since neither will be receiving more glucose if not fat is replaced.

If you were in Ketosis and you lost it lean on the intermittent fasting avoiding breakfast and lunch and April no later your feeding window in this way your organism will understand that you must take the ketosis to keep it.

Accompanying the keto diet with the intermittent breakfast from the beginning accelerates the process of ketosis allowed your body to catch up within the first 24 to 48 hours.

Fatty fasting consists of eating in your 8-hour window only healthy foods such as avocado, coconut oil, salmon, tilapia and other seafood and avoiding carbohydrates.

3 STEP

INCREASE YOUR PHYSICAL ACTIVITY

◆ ◆ ◆

One of the best ways to speed up ketosis is by getting your body to consume stored glucose more quickly and for that.

It is necessary to increase your level of physical activity even more if you have a sedentary lifestyle. To achieve this, increase your daily routine by 20 minutes of intense physical exercise, such as a CrossFit Spinning session or even a short run.

The important thing is that you activate your body's need to burn the glycogen hidden in the muscles so that it has no choice but to start burning the fat.

A major boost to reach ketosis will come if you exercise before breakfast so that your body can more quickly extract all the stored glycogen for energy.

Also remember not to get stuck in your physical activity climb stairs walk a little at home dance a little everything that allows you to accelerate the process of burning glucose is welcome to accelerate the ketosis.

4 STEP

DRINK 2 TO 3 LITERS
OF WATER PER DAY

◆ ◆ ◆

Drinking 3 liters of water a day helps you enter ketosis in a healthy way and maintain it and helps you stay hydrated.

When your carbohydrate intake decreases the body no longer has the same support system to retain water.

Since carbohydrates are the main source where you stay and this can make you dehydrate quickly.

Under dehydration the body stops its functions including the liver stops performing certain tasks such as ketosis to take over the support of the kidneys and help it process and remove toxins from the body that the kidney is responsible for removing.

If the liver is taking care of other functions I can no longer process ketones so it stops the fat burning process so dehydration can get you out of ketosis even prevent it from entering it.

To avoid dehydration, the ideal is to maintain proper hydration with electrolyte replacement but without resorting to energy drinks.

What you should do is drink a lot of water and add a pinch of salt to replenish your lost sodium levels.

A person weighing approximately 72 kg needs to consume about 80 ounces (2.37 l) of water per day, which is approximately 2 liters of water.

But you don't need to drink all of it at once, you can alternate it throughout the day and thus facilitate your body's thermoregulation function.

5 STEP

INCREASE YOUR
BLACK COFFEE INTAKE

◆ ◆ ◆

A sugar- and milk-free coffee is a magic substance that accelerates the process of ketosis and its effect helps to avoid the feeling of hunger, since it reduces the amount of the hormone ghrelin in the blood.

Better known as the hunger hormone which will cause your hunger levels to decrease and your half-day cravings to decrease as well.

Even before breakfast is ideal to reduce your feeling of hunger and take it a couple of times a day.

It is an excellent support tool for achieving ketosis by helping you to maintain satiety and keep your 20 gram carbohydrate diet.

If you don't like coffee you can drink tea but remember that it should be without sugars of any kind even without sweeteners and of course without milk.

6 STEP

AVOID SNACKS, EVEN KETO SNACKS

◆ ◆ ◆

I t is very common to feel hungry at any time when starting a ketogenic diet.

Well, your body was used to being full of high-sugar carbs, but fats are not so good at taking away the craving for something sweet.

But it is vital that to achieve ketosis in 24 hours you stop snacking outside the meal.

Even if they are ketogenic, some famous snacks can also provide many carbohydrates if you go over the top.

Many nuts like cashews and peanuts can provide all the carbohydrate load allowed in the diet.

And even if you get over it by eating a couple of handfuls of them to make a partnership, if you add the charges you've already consumed, you can say goodbye to ketosis.

It is therefore essential that you stop snacking even if you find it compatible with the ketogenic diet at least for the first 24 hours while you manage to get to ketosis.

7 STEP

BREAKING THE CARBOHYDRATE-FREE FASTING

◆ ◆ ◆

Starting your feeding window without ingesting carbohydrates is another way to give your body a lift towards ketosis your body will always be looking for the easiest option to get energy and if you give it some carbohydrates from the first moment that is the first thing it will process.

So beat the process and force it into ketosis by providing only fat and some protein from the moment you open your feeding window. One option is to start your meal with eggs or a tuna salad.

8 STEP

CONSUME OIL MCT

Triglyceride-containing oils with the medium chain OMCT are a good support for ketosis, since it is the triglycerides and fatty acids that are broken down in the liver to produce ketones.

These oils can be obtained naturally through the consumption of coconut oil or from the animal kingdom such as butter, but there are also processed products.

Specifically to give you the MCT contribution that requires these can be found in online stores or in your favorite Keto store.

9 STEP

START THE KETOGENIC DIET AT THE WEEKEND

◆ ◆ ◆

Often a drastic change in diet can lead to minor health problems as the body gets used to the change.

Especially when it comes to carbohydrate reduction some of them can be dizziness nausea physical weakness that hinders their cognitive process these symptoms are known as the keto flu.

They are usually present at the beginning of the process to avoid feeling bad during working hours or when it requires their highest concentration. It is advisable to start the ketogenic diet in a weekend.

Starting on Friday and continue with two days off from adaptation another point to consider is to start a change of diet requires your greatest attention and willpower so it is easier to stick to the plan is at home.

Where Keto food is within reach and you don't run the risk of being tempted with snacks and full of carbohydrates.

Even if your family doesn't stick to the same eating plan, it will still be easier to start at home because you can explain your goal to them and ask for their support to help you succeed in those first hours of your ketogenic diet.

Whether you encourage or away from any dangerous food for your ketosis but do not believe it is always easier to start and maintain a diet and have the support of those who live

With you.

10 STEP

SLEEPS 8 TO 10 HOURS A DAY

◆ ◆ ◆

During sleep the body is fasting which in turn allows blood glucose levels to drop

If you sleep 8-10 hours a day this will be a net fasting time for you so it didn't seem so forced to keep fasting a few more hours if you are practicing intermittent fasting.

Another advantage of sleeping long enough and sleeping well is that your cortisol level also drops.

Cortisol is the stress hormone and a short, unstable sleep can cause your blood insulin levels to rise and this will not allow you to achieve ketosis.

To reach ketosis in 24 hours or to resume the count of the number of carbohydrates you are consuming per day you could be

Exceeding the limit it must consume reminds many Vegetables also provide carbohydrates.

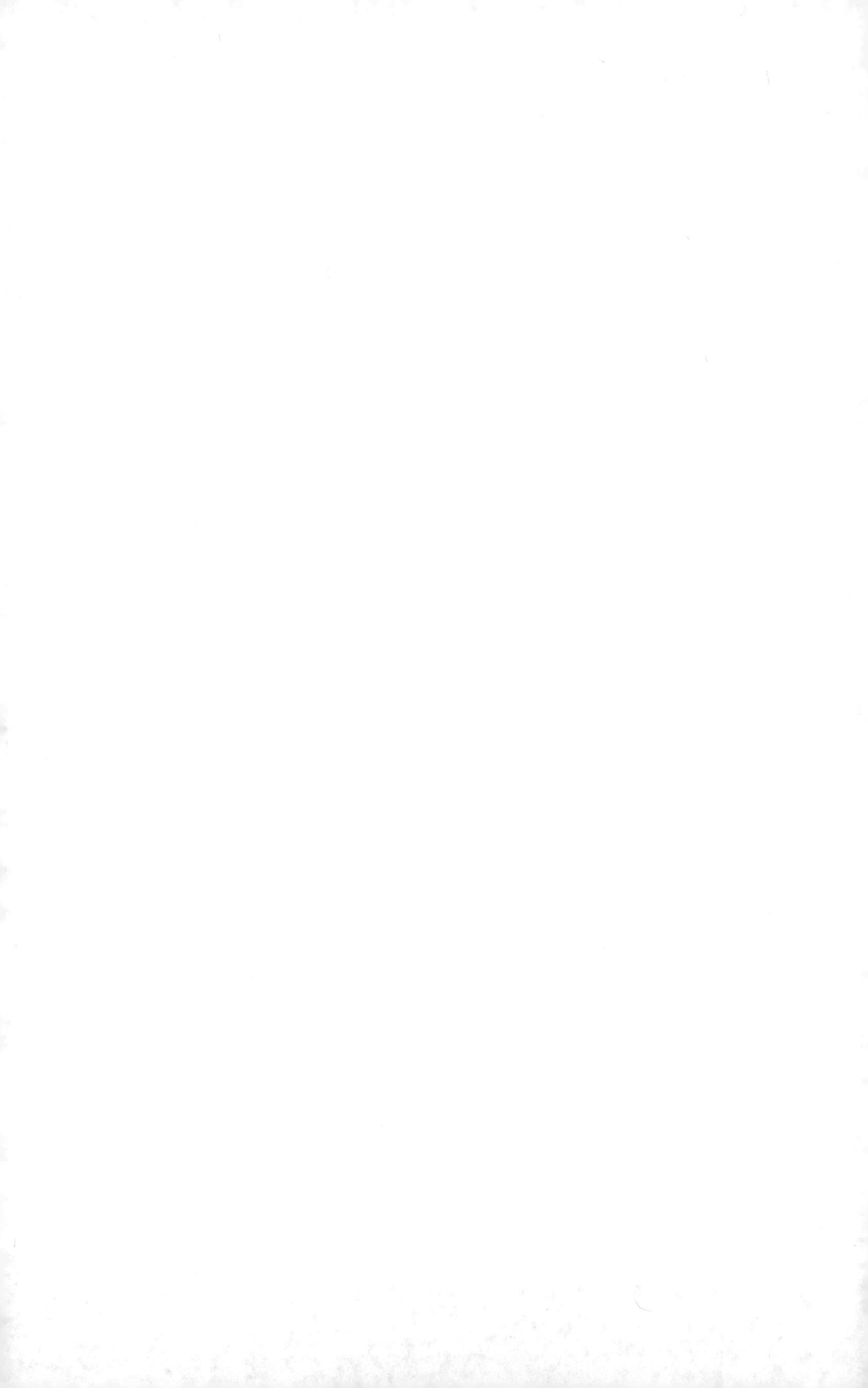